PRITIKIN DIET COOKBOOK

guide and delicious recipes for managing your weight and diabetes meal plan for a healthy living

Alex kava

Copyright

No part of this publication may be reproduced, distributed, or transmitted in any form or by any means, including photocopying, recording, or other electronic or mechanical methods, without the prior written permission of the publisher, except in the case of brief quotations embodied in critical reviews and certain other noncommercial uses permitted by copyright law.

Table of Contents

Introduction

Meet Sarah, a culinary enthusiast with a passion for crafting nutritious and delectable meals. Armed with nothing more than the title of the **"Pritikin Diet Cookbook,"** Sarah has transformed her kitchen into a haven of health and flavor.

With an intuitive understanding of the Pritikin Diet principles, Sarah navigates the art of combining whole, unprocessed foods, lean proteins, and high-fiber carbohydrates effortlessly. The cookbook serves as her guide, inspiring a culinary journey that revolves around fresh ingredients and mindful preparation.

Sarah's kitchen buzzes with activity as she seamlessly executes vibrant salads, hearty main courses, and guilt-free desserts from the cookbook's pages. Her meals are a testament to the belief that eating well need not compromise on taste. Each dish she prepares is not just a recipe; it's a manifestation of the Pritikin philosophy— where wholesome choices contribute not only to weight management but also to overall health and well-being.

What sets Sarah apart is not just her ability to follow recipes but her understanding of the underlying principles. The Pritikin Diet Cookbook isn't merely a collection of instructions for her; it's a gateway to a lifestyle marked by balance and sustainability. As Sarah shares her nutritious creations with friends and family, the cookbook becomes a source of inspiration, sparking conversations about mindful eating and the impact of food choices on our health.

For Sarah, the Pritikin Diet Cookbook isn't just a book; it's a culinary companion that has transformed the way she approaches food. Her kitchen is now a space where health and flavor coexist harmoniously, thanks to her innate ability to translate cookbook wisdom into wholesome, delicious meals that nourish both body and soul.

Chapter 1: Introduction to the Pritikin Diet

The Pritikin Diet is a dietary approach that gained popularity for its emphasis on promoting heart health and overall well-being through a combination of a low-fat, high-fiber diet and regular exercise. Developed by Nathan Pritikin in the late 1970s, the Pritikin Diet is rooted in the belief that a plant-based, whole-foods diet, coupled with a physically active lifestyle, can significantly reduce the risk of heart disease and other chronic illnesses.

Nathan Pritikin, a nutritionist and longevity researcher, was motivated by his own health struggles and a desire to find a sustainable and natural way to prevent and treat cardiovascular issues. His approach to nutrition focuses on incorporating primarily whole, unprocessed foods and limiting the intake of saturated fats and cholesterol, which are often associated with heart disease.

The core principles of the Pritikin Diet include:

1. Low-Fat, High-Fiber Foods: The diet encourages the consumption of foods that are naturally low in fat and high in fiber. This includes a variety of fruits, vegetables, whole grains, legumes, and lean protein sources.

2. Minimizing Processed Foods: Highly processed foods, which often contain added sugars, unhealthy fats, and excess salt, are discouraged on the Pritikin Diet. Instead, the emphasis is on choosing whole, natural foods that provide essential nutrients without the drawbacks associated with processed products.

3. Limiting Animal Products: While not strictly vegetarian, the Pritikin Diet advocates for a reduction in the intake of animal products, especially those high in saturated fats. Lean sources of protein, such as fish and poultry, are recommended over red meat.

4.   Exercise: In   addition   to   dietary recommendations, the Pritikin Diet emphasizes regular physical activity as a crucial component of a healthy lifestyle. Exercise is seen as a complement to the dietary guidelines, contributing to cardiovascular health and overall well-being.

5. Weight Management: The Pritikin Diet is often associated with weight management and can be effective for those looking to lose weight or maintain a healthy weight. The focus on nutrient-dense, low-calorie foods can support individuals in achieving and sustaining a healthy body weight.

The Pritikin Diet has been studied for its potential health benefits, with research suggesting positive effects on cholesterol levels, blood pressure, and overall cardiovascular health. However, it's important to note that individual responses to the diet may vary, and consulting with a healthcare professional before making significant dietary changes is advisable, especially for individuals with pre-existing health conditions.

The Pritikin Diet promotes a plant-based, whole-foods approach to nutrition, combined with regular exercise, as a means to enhance heart health and overall well-being. While it may not be suitable for everyone, its principles align with broader recommendations for a healthy lifestyle, emphasizing the importance of a balanced diet and physical activity in promoting long-term health.

The Pritikin Approach to Health

The Pritikin Diet, rooted in the pioneering work of Nathan Pritikin, represents more than just a dietary regimen; it embodies a comprehensive approach to health and well-being. Nathan Pritikin, a nutritionist and longevity researcher, introduced this approach in the late 1970s with a vision to combat cardiovascular diseases and promote overall vitality through a combination of nutrition, exercise, and lifestyle modifications.

The Core Principles of the Pritikin Approach:

1. Dietary Emphasis on Heart Health:

The cornerstone of the Pritikin Approach lies in its dietary principles, meticulously designed to promote heart health. The diet advocates for a shift toward whole, unprocessed foods that are naturally low in fat and high in fiber. Fruits, vegetables, whole grains, legumes, and lean protein sources take center stage, while the intake of saturated fats and cholesterol is limited. This dietary focus aligns with the goal of reducing the risk of heart disease, a leading cause of mortality worldwide.

2. Minimizing Processed and Refined Foods:

Recognizing the detrimental effects of processed and refined foods, the Pritikin Approach encourages individuals to steer clear of such items. Highly processed foods often contain excessive sugars, unhealthy fats, and additives linked to various health issues. By advocating for whole, nutrient-dense foods, the approach aims to provide essential nutrients without the drawbacks associated with processed alternatives.

3. Balancing Animal Products:

While not strictly vegetarian, the Pritikin Approach suggests a moderation in the consumption of animal products, particularly those high in saturated fats. The emphasis is on choosing lean protein sources such as fish and poultry over red meat. This balanced approach aims to maintain adequate protein intake while minimizing the potential adverse effects associated with excessive consumption of certain animal products.

4. Holistic Perspective on Exercise:

In addition to dietary guidelines, the Pritikin Approach places significant importance on regular physical activity. Exercise is viewed as an integral component of overall health, contributing not only to cardiovascular fitness but also to weight management and mental well-being. The philosophy emphasizes that a sedentary lifestyle can contribute to various health issues and that incorporating regular physical activity is essential for a holistic approach to health.

5. Weight Management and Beyond:

Beyond its association with heart health, the Pritikin Approach is often embraced for its effectiveness in weight management. By promoting a diet rich in nutrient-dense, low-calorie foods and encouraging regular exercise, the approach supports individuals in achieving and maintaining a healthy body weight. Moreover, the benefits extend beyond weight, encompassing improved energy levels, enhanced mood, and a reduced risk of various chronic diseases.

The Pritikin Approach to Health, encapsulated by the Pritikin Diet, offers a holistic framework that goes beyond mere dietary guidelines. It embodies a lifestyle philosophy that underscores the interconnectedness of nutrition, exercise, and overall well-being. Rooted in scientific research and decades of practical application, the Pritikin Approach continues to inspire individuals to take charge of their health by making informed choices that foster longevity and vitality.

The Science Behind the Pritikin Diet

The Pritikin Diet, a renowned approach to nutrition, is underpinned by a robust scientific foundation that extends beyond popular diet trends. Developed by Nathan Pritikin, a pioneer in the field of nutrition and longevity, the Pritikin Diet is grounded in scientific principles aimed at promoting heart health, reducing the risk of chronic diseases, and optimizing overall well-being.

Understanding the Science Behind the Pritikin Diet:

1. Cholesterol and Heart Health:

At the heart of the Pritikin Diet is a focus on cholesterol reduction, a critical factor in preventing cardiovascular diseases. Scientific studies consistently demonstrate the correlation between high cholesterol levels and increased risk of heart-related issues. By advocating for a diet low in saturated and trans fats, the Pritikin approach aims to lower blood cholesterol levels, fostering cardiovascular health.

2. Fiber-Rich Nutrition:

The Pritikin Diet places a strong emphasis on consuming foods high in dietary fiber. Scientifically, dietary fiber has been linked to various health benefits, including improved digestion, better blood sugar control, and a reduced risk of heart disease. Whole grains, fruits, and vegetables, key components of the Pritikin Diet, contribute to increased fiber intake, supporting both digestive health and overall well-being.

3. Impact on Blood Pressure:

Research indicates a close relationship between dietary patterns and blood pressure regulation. The Pritikin Diet, rich in potassium, calcium, and magnesium from fruits and vegetables, has been shown to have a positive impact on blood pressure levels. The combination of nutrient-dense foods and reduced sodium intake aligns with scientific recommendations for maintaining healthy blood pressure.

4. Weight Management and Metabolic Health:

Scientific evidence consistently supports the role of diet in weight management and metabolic health. The Pritikin Diet, with its emphasis on whole, low-calorie, and nutrient-dense foods, aligns with principles that facilitate weight loss and the maintenance of a healthy weight. This, in turn, contributes to improved metabolic markers and a reduced risk of obesity-related conditions.

5. Exercise Physiology:

The integration of regular exercise into the Pritikin Approach is grounded in the science of exercise physiology. Scientific research demonstrates that physical activity not only contributes to cardiovascular fitness but also plays a crucial role in weight management, mental health, and overall longevity. The Pritikin philosophy recognizes the synergistic effects of combining a healthful diet with regular exercise for optimal well-being.

The Pritikin Diet stands out not only for its practical approach but also for its scientific rigor. Rooted in the understanding of how specific dietary choices impact physiological processes, the Pritikin Diet aligns with evidence-based recommendations for cardiovascular health, weight management, and overall longevity. By embracing the science behind optimal nutrition, the Pritikin Diet continues to empower individuals to make informed choices that resonate with their health goals, translating scientific knowledge into practical and sustainable lifestyle changes.

Benefits of the Pritikin Diet

The Pritikin Diet, renowned for its holistic approach to nutrition and lifestyle, offers a myriad of health benefits that extend beyond mere weight management. Developed by Nathan Pritikin, this dietary approach has garnered attention for its potential to promote optimal health and well-being. Let's delve into the key benefits of the Pritikin Diet.

1. Heart Health:

A central tenet of the Pritikin Diet is its focus on heart health. By emphasizing a diet low in saturated and trans fats, and rich in whole, plant-based foods, the Pritikin approach aims to lower cholesterol levels and reduce the risk of cardiovascular diseases. Numerous studies have supported the positive impact of the Pritikin Diet on factors such as blood pressure and lipid profiles, contributing to a healthier heart.

2. Weight Management:

The Pritikin Diet is recognized for its effectiveness in weight management. The emphasis on nutrient-dense, low-calorie foods, coupled with regular exercise, provides a balanced approach to achieving and maintaining a healthy weight. This not only supports aesthetic goals but also contributes to the prevention of obesity-related conditions, such as type 2 diabetes and metabolic syndrome.

3. Blood Sugar Control:

The Pritikin Diet, rich in complex carbohydrates from whole grains, fruits, and vegetables, can contribute to better blood sugar control. The inclusion of fiber helps regulate glucose absorption, reducing the risk of insulin resistance and type 2 diabetes. Scientific evidence suggests that adopting the Pritikin approach may positively impact glycemic control and insulin sensitivity.

4. Reduced Inflammation:

Chronic inflammation is implicated in various health issues, including heart disease and autoimmune conditions. The Pritikin Diet, with its emphasis on anti-inflammatory foods such as fruits, vegetables, and omega-3 fatty acids, may contribute to a reduction in inflammation. This anti-inflammatory effect is crucial for overall health and may play a role in preventing and managing chronic diseases.

5. Improved Mental Well-being:

The Pritikin Diet is not solely focused on physical health; it also acknowledges the intricate connection between nutrition and mental well-being. Nutrient-rich foods that support brain health, combined with regular exercise, can positively influence mood and cognitive function. The Pritikin approach advocates for a holistic lifestyle that fosters mental clarity and emotional balance.

6. Longevity and Quality of Life:

Beyond immediate health benefits, adhering to the Pritikin Diet is associated with longevity and an enhanced quality of life. By addressing key factors linked to aging, such as heart health, weight management, and inflammation, individuals following the Pritikin approach may experience a more vibrant and active lifestyle as they age.

The Pritikin Diet offers a comprehensive approach to health, presenting a wealth of benefits that extend across various facets of well-being. By embracing a diet rich in whole, unprocessed foods, coupled with regular exercise, individuals can unlock the potential for improved cardiovascular health, sustainable weight management, better blood sugar control, reduced inflammation, enhanced mental well-being, and a longer, more fulfilling life. As individuals explore the Pritikin Diet, they embark on a journey towards holistic health and vitality.

Chapter 2: The Essentials of the Pritikin Diet

The Pritikin Diet is a lifestyle and dietary approach developed by Nathan Pritikin in the 1970s. It emphasizes a low-fat, high-fiber, plant-based eating pattern to promote overall health and prevent chronic diseases. The core philosophy behind the Pritikin Diet is to prioritize whole, nutrient-dense foods while minimizing the intake of processed and high-fat options. Here are some essential aspects of the Pritikin Diet:

1. Whole Foods Emphasis:

The foundation of the Pritikin Diet is built on whole, unprocessed foods. This includes fruits, vegetables, whole grains, legumes, and lean proteins. Whole foods are rich in essential nutrients and fiber, which contribute to satiety and overall well-being.

2. Low-Fat Approach:

The Pritikin Diet advocates for a low-fat intake, particularly saturated and trans fats. By choosing lean protein sources, such as skinless poultry, fish, and plant-based proteins, and limiting added fats and oils, individuals following this diet aim to reduce their risk of cardiovascular diseases.

3. High Fiber Intake:

Fiber is a crucial component of the Pritikin Diet. It aids in digestion, helps control blood sugar levels, and contributes to a feeling of fullness. Fruits, vegetables, whole grains, and legumes are excellent sources of dietary fiber and are encouraged as part of every meal.

4. Limiting Refined Sugar and Processed Foods:

Processed foods, especially those high in refined sugar and unhealthy fats, are discouraged on the Pritikin Diet. These items contribute empty calories and can lead to weight gain and other health issues. Instead, individuals are encouraged to satisfy their sweet tooth with naturally sweet fruits.

5. Balanced Macronutrients:

While the emphasis is on reducing fat intake, the Pritikin Diet promotes a balanced intake of macronutrients. Carbohydrates, proteins, and fats are all included in the diet, but the focus is on choosing the right sources and proportions to support overall health.

6. Regular Exercise:

The Pritikin Diet is often coupled with a commitment to regular physical activity. Exercise is considered a vital component of a healthy lifestyle and complements the dietary principles of the Pritikin approach. Both aerobic and strength training exercises are recommended.

7. Education and Lifestyle Changes:

Beyond the immediate dietary guidelines, the Pritikin Diet encourages individuals to educate themselves about nutrition and make sustainable lifestyle changes. This includes mindful eating, stress management, and adopting healthier habits that extend beyond the dining table.

8. Medical Supervision:

Individuals with existing health conditions or those considering a significant dietary change, especially if it involves any form of caloric restriction, should seek guidance from healthcare professionals. The Pritikin Diet may be particularly beneficial for those with cardiovascular concerns, but personalized advice is essential.

The Pritikin Diet promotes a holistic lifestyle centered around whole, nutrient-dense foods, regular exercise, and mindful living. While its primary focus is cardiovascular health, the principles of the Pritikin Diet align with broader goals of overall well-being and disease prevention.

The Pritikin Food Pyramid

The Pritikin Food Pyramid is a visual representation of the recommended food choices within the Pritikin Diet, emphasizing a plant-based, low-fat approach to nutrition. This pyramid provides a clear guide for individuals seeking to adopt the Pritikin lifestyle and make informed choices about their dietary intake. Here are the essential components of the Pritikin Food Pyramid:

1. Base: Fruits and Vegetables

At the base of the Pritikin Food Pyramid are fruits and vegetables. These plant-based foods form the foundation of a Pritikin-friendly diet due to their rich nutrient content, including vitamins, minerals, and antioxidants. A variety of colorful fruits and vegetables are recommended to ensure a diverse range of nutrients.

2. Whole Grains

The next tier of the pyramid consists of whole grains such as oats, brown rice, quinoa, and whole wheat bread. Whole grains provide complex carbohydrates and fiber, promoting satiety and supporting digestive health. They also contribute essential nutrients like B vitamins and iron.

3. Legumes and Beans

Legumes and beans, including lentils, chickpeas, and black beans, occupy a significant portion of the

Pritikin Food Pyramid. These plant-based protein sources are not only low in fat but also high in fiber, making them an essential component for those following the Pritikin Diet.

4. Lean Proteins

Lean proteins, such as skinless poultry, fish, and plant-based protein alternatives like tofu and tempeh, are included in moderate amounts. These protein sources are preferred over high-fat options and provide essential amino acids necessary for bodily functions.

5. Low-Fat Dairy or Dairy Alternatives

The Pritikin Diet allows for low-fat dairy products or dairy alternatives. These include options like skim milk, low-fat yogurt, and plant-based milk substitutes. Calcium and vitamin D from these sources contribute to bone health.

6. Nuts and Seeds (Moderation)

While high in healthy fats, nuts and seeds are included in moderation on the Pritikin Food Pyramid. They offer beneficial nutrients, including omega-3 fatty acids and various vitamins and minerals. Portion control is emphasized to manage calorie intake.

7. Herbs, Spices, and Flavorings

Herbs, spices, and flavorings are encouraged to enhance the taste of meals without the need for excessive salt, sugar, or added fats. This not only adds variety to the diet but also aligns with the Pritikin philosophy of minimizing processed and refined ingredients.

8. Limit Sweets and Added Sugars

Sweets and added sugars are placed at the top of the pyramid, indicating that they should be consumed sparingly. The Pritikin Diet advises against the excessive intake of sugary foods and beverages, promoting the use of natural sweeteners found in fruits instead.

9. Limit Fats and Oils

Fats and oils occupy the smallest section at the top of the pyramid, reinforcing the Pritikin Diet's emphasis on reducing overall fat intake. Healthy fats, such as those from olive oil and avocados, are recommended in moderation.

10. Stay Hydrated

While not explicitly depicted on the pyramid, staying hydrated is a crucial aspect of the Pritikin Diet. Water is the preferred beverage, and individuals are encouraged to limit the consumption of sugary drinks and alcohol.

The Pritikin Food Pyramid serves as a practical tool for individuals looking to align their dietary choices with the principles of the Pritikin Diet. It promotes a balanced and nutrient-dense approach to eating, with an emphasis on plant-based foods and mindful choices for overall health and well-being.

Whole Foods, Plant–Based Nutrition

The Pritikin Diet places a strong emphasis on whole foods, particularly those derived from plant sources. This plant-based approach to nutrition is rooted in the belief that a diet rich in fruits, vegetables, whole grains, and legumes can contribute to overall health and well-being. Here are the key essentials of whole foods, plant-based nutrition within the context of the Pritikin Diet:

1. Abundance of Fruits and Vegetables:

A cornerstone of the Pritikin Diet is the abundant consumption of fruits and vegetables. These foods are rich in vitamins, minerals, antioxidants, and fiber, which collectively support immune function, aid digestion, and contribute to heart health. A colorful variety of fruits and vegetables is recommended to ensure a diverse range of nutrients.

2. Whole Grains for Sustained Energy:

Whole grains, such as brown rice, quinoa, oats, and whole wheat, are integral to the Pritikin Diet. Unlike refined grains, whole grains contain the bran, germ, and endosperm, providing fiber, essential nutrients, and a sustained release of energy. These grains are central to promoting satiety and supporting a healthy metabolism.

3. Plant-Based Proteins:

The Pritikin Diet encourages the inclusion of plant-based protein sources such as legumes, beans, tofu, tempeh, and edamame. These alternatives provide essential amino acids without the saturated fats often associated with animal-based proteins. Plant-based proteins are also rich in fiber, aiding in digestive health.

4. Healthy Fats from Plant Sources:

While the Pritikin Diet is low in overall fat content, it recognizes the importance of including healthy fats from plant sources. Avocados, nuts, seeds, and olive oil are recommended in moderation for their contributions to heart health and overall well-being.

5. Minimization of Processed Foods:

The Pritikin Diet advises against the consumption of highly processed foods. Processed foods often contain added sugars, unhealthy fats, and excess sodium. Instead, the focus is on whole, minimally processed foods to maximize nutrient intake and minimize the intake of empty calories.

6. Emphasis on Fiber:

Plant-based foods are naturally high in dietary fiber, a key component of the Pritikin Diet. Fiber not only supports digestive health but also contributes to a feeling of fullness, helping to manage weight. Additionally, fiber has been associated with improved cholesterol levels and a reduced risk of heart disease.

7. Hydration with Water:

Water is the beverage of choice in the Pritikin Diet. Staying well-hydrated supports overall health, aids digestion, and helps regulate appetite. Sugary drinks and excessive caffeine are discouraged in favor of water to maintain optimal hydration.

8. Focus on Nutrient Density:

The Pritikin Diet promotes the concept of nutrient density, emphasizing foods that provide a high concentration of essential nutrients relative to their calorie content. This approach ensures that individuals receive the maximum nutritional benefit from their food choices.

9. Individualized Approach:

While the Pritikin Diet has general principles, it recognizes that individual nutritional needs may vary. It encourages individuals to listen to their bodies, make mindful food choices, and adopt a sustainable and personalized approach to plant-based nutrition.

The Pritikin Diet's emphasis on whole foods and plant-based nutrition aligns with a growing body of research suggesting the health benefits of such dietary patterns. By prioritizing nutrient-dense, plant-derived foods, the Pritikin Diet offers a roadmap for individuals seeking to optimize their health through a wholesome and sustainable approach to nutrition.

Lean Proteins and Healthy Fats

The Pritikin Diet is a renowned approach to healthy living that focuses on a balanced and sustainable way of eating. Developed by Nathan Pritikin in the 1970s, this diet emphasizes whole foods, particularly those that are low in fat and sodium, to promote overall health and well-being. One of the key components of the Pritikin Diet is the inclusion of lean proteins and healthy fats, which play crucial roles in maintaining a balanced and nutritious eating plan.

Lean Proteins: The Foundation of Pritikin Diet

Lean proteins are an essential component of the Pritikin Diet, providing the body with the necessary building blocks for muscle development, repair, and overall cellular function. Unlike many traditional diets that might encourage high consumption of red meats and processed meats, the Pritikin Diet encourages the intake of lean protein sources, such as:

1. Fish: Fatty fish like salmon, mackerel, and trout are rich in omega-3 fatty acids, which contribute to heart health. These fish are favored over those with higher mercury content, promoting both protein intake and cardiovascular well-being.

2. Skinless Poultry: Chicken and turkey without the skin are excellent sources of lean protein. These options provide essential amino acids without the added saturated fats found in the skin.

3. Plant-Based Proteins: Legumes, beans, lentils, and tofu are integral parts of the Pritikin Diet, offering plant-based protein options that are low in fat and high in fiber. They contribute to satiety and help maintain a healthy weight.

4. Lean Cuts of Meat: If red meat is consumed, opting for lean cuts such as sirloin or tenderloin can provide protein without excessive saturated fat content.

Healthy Fats: A Balancing Act

While many diets discourage the intake of fats, the Pritikin Diet recognizes the importance of incorporating healthy fats into the daily eating routine. Healthy fats are crucial for various bodily functions, including brain health, hormone production, and the absorption of fat-soluble vitamins. The Pritikin Diet encourages the consumption of:

1. Nuts and Seeds: Almonds, walnuts, flaxseeds, and chia seeds are rich in omega-3 fatty acids, fiber, and antioxidants. They serve as healthy snacks or additions to meals.

2. Avocado: This creamy fruit is a great source of monounsaturated fats, which are heart-healthy fats that can help lower bad cholesterol levels.

3. Olive Oil: Extra virgin olive oil is a staple in the Pritikin Diet, providing monounsaturated fats that are beneficial for heart health. It is used in cooking and as a dressing for salads.

4. Fatty Fish: In addition to being a lean protein source, fatty fish like salmon and mackerel contribute essential omega-3 fatty acids to the diet, supporting cardiovascular health and brain function.

Portion Control and Overall Lifestyle

In addition to focusing on specific food choices, the Pritikin Diet emphasizes portion control and an overall healthy lifestyle. By adopting mindful eating habits and engaging in regular physical activity, individuals following the Pritikin Diet aim to achieve and maintain a healthy weight, reduce the risk of chronic diseases, and improve overall well-being.

The Pritikin Diet places a strong emphasis on the importance of lean proteins and healthy fats. By making informed choices about the sources and amounts of these nutrients, individuals can create a well-rounded and sustainable eating plan that supports their health and fitness goals.

Understanding Fiber and Its Role in Weight Management

The Pritikin Diet is renowned for its holistic approach to health, and a key element of this regimen is a focus on dietary fiber. Fiber is a crucial component that plays a significant role in weight management, digestive health, and overall well-being. In the context of the Pritikin Diet, understanding the importance of fiber and incorporating it into the daily eating plan is fundamental for achieving and maintaining a healthy lifestyle.

The Role of Fiber in Weight Management

1. Satiety and Reduced Caloric Intake:

Dietary fiber, found in fruits, vegetables, whole grains, and legumes, adds bulk to meals, promoting a feeling of fullness. This increased satiety can lead to reduced overall caloric intake, supporting weight management by helping individuals avoid excessive snacking and overeating.

2. Slow Digestion and Blood Sugar Regulation:

Soluble fiber, prevalent in foods like oats, beans, and fruits, slows down the digestion and absorption of nutrients. This can help regulate blood sugar levels, preventing spikes and crashes that may contribute to cravings for sugary or high-calorie foods.

3. Improved Gut Health:

Insoluble fiber, found in foods like whole grains and vegetables, adds bulk to stools and aids in regular bowel movements. This promotes a healthy digestive system, preventing constipation and promoting optimal nutrient absorption.

Pritikin Diet-Friendly Fiber Sources

1. Whole Grains: Foods like brown rice, quinoa, and whole wheat provide a rich source of dietary fiber. These grains can be incorporated into meals, adding nutritional value and promoting feelings of fullness.

2. Fruits and Vegetables: The Pritikin Diet encourages the consumption of a variety of colorful fruits and vegetables, as they are naturally high in fiber, vitamins, and antioxidants. Berries, apples, broccoli, and spinach are excellent choices.

3. Legumes: Beans, lentils, and peas are not only rich in protein but also high in fiber. They serve as versatile ingredients in soups, stews, salads, and other Pritikin Diet-friendly dishes.

4. Nuts and Seeds: Almonds, chia seeds, and flaxseeds are not only excellent sources of healthy fats but also contribute fiber to the diet. They can be incorporated into meals, snacks, or added to smoothies for an extra nutritional boost.

Practical Tips for Increasing Fiber Intake

1. Gradual Incorporation: It's advisable to gradually increase fiber intake to allow the digestive system to adjust. Sudden increases may lead to bloating or discomfort.

2. Hydration: Adequate water intake is essential when consuming more fiber, as it helps prevent constipation and supports the movement of fiber through the digestive tract.

3. Variety is Key: The Pritikin Diet encourages a diverse range of fiber sources to ensure a broad spectrum of nutrients. Eating a variety of fruits, vegetables, whole grains, and legumes contributes to a balanced and satisfying diet.

Incorporating an ample amount of fiber into the Pritikin Diet is a cornerstone of this approach to healthy living. By understanding the role of fiber in weight management and overall well-being, individuals can make informed choices about the foods they consume, fostering a sustainable and health-conscious lifestyle.

Chapter 3: Meal Planning for Diabetes Management

Managing diabetes effectively involves making thoughtful and informed choices about what and when to eat. Meal planning plays a crucial role in controlling blood sugar levels, maintaining a healthy weight, and preventing complications associated with diabetes. Here's a comprehensive guide to help you navigate meal planning for diabetes management:

Understanding the Basics:

1. Carbohydrate Counting:

  - **Why it matters:** Carbohydrates have a direct impact on blood sugar levels. Monitoring and managing carbohydrate intake is crucial for controlling diabetes.

- **How to do it:** Learn to read food labels, measure serving sizes, and understand the carbohydrate content of different foods.

2. Glycemic Index (GI):

- **What it is:** The GI measures how quickly a food raises blood sugar levels. Low-GI foods are digested more slowly and have a smaller impact on blood sugar.

- **How to use it:** Choose mostly low-GI foods like whole grains, legumes, and non-starchy vegetables to help stabilize blood sugar.

Building a Balanced Plate:

3. Portion Control:

- **Why it's important:** Controlling portion sizes helps manage calorie intake, which is essential for weight management and blood sugar control.

- **Tips:** Use smaller plates, measure portions, and be mindful of portion sizes to avoid overeating.

4. Protein Intake:

- **Role in diabetes management:** Protein helps with satiety, supports muscle health, and has a minimal impact on blood sugar levels.

- **Sources:** Include lean proteins like poultry, fish, tofu, legumes, and low-fat dairy in your meals.

5. Healthy Fats:

- **Importance:** Healthy fats contribute to heart health and can help stabilize blood sugar levels.

- **Sources:** Include sources of monounsaturated and polyunsaturated fats such as avocados, nuts, seeds, and olive oil.

Planning Smart Meals:

6. Regular Meal Timing:

- **Consistency matters:** Eating meals and snacks at consistent times helps regulate blood sugar levels.

- **Avoid skipping meals:** Skipping meals can lead to blood sugar fluctuations. Plan for regular, balanced meals.

7. Fiber-Rich Foods:

- **Benefits:** Fiber aids in digestion, helps control blood sugar levels, and promotes a feeling of fullness.

- **Sources:** Include whole grains, fruits, vegetables, and legumes to increase fiber intake.

8. Limiting Sugary and Processed Foods:

- **Why it's crucial:** Processed foods and those high in added sugars can cause rapid spikes in blood sugar.

- **Alternatives:** Opt for whole, unprocessed foods and use natural sweeteners in moderation.

Special Considerations:

9. Individualized Approach:

- **Consult a dietitian:** Work with a healthcare professional or a registered dietitian to create a personalized meal plan based on your individual needs, preferences, and lifestyle.

10. Monitoring and Adjusting:

- **Regular blood sugar monitoring:** Keep track of your blood sugar levels to understand how different foods affect you. Adjust your meal plan accordingly.

11. Incorporating Physical Activity:

- **Role in diabetes management:** Regular exercise helps control blood sugar, improves insulin sensitivity, and supports overall health.

- **Timing of meals and exercise:** Coordinate your meals and snacks with your exercise routine for optimal results.

Effective meal planning is a cornerstone of successful diabetes management. By adopting a balanced and individualized approach, incorporating nutrient-dense foods, and staying mindful of portion sizes, you can create a meal plan that promotes stable blood sugar levels and overall well-being. Always consult with your healthcare team for personalized advice and adjustments to your diabetes management plan.

Diabetes and Diet: A Holistic Approach

Living with diabetes requires a holistic approach that goes beyond medication and includes a careful consideration of dietary choices. Meal planning plays a central role in managing diabetes effectively, offering a powerful tool to control blood sugar levels, maintain a healthy weight, and improve overall well-being. Here's a guide to adopting a holistic approach to diabetes management through mindful meal planning:

Understanding the Relationship Between Diabetes and Diet:

1. The Impact of Carbohydrates:

- **Balancing Act:** Carbohydrates significantly affect blood sugar levels. Understanding the types of carbohydrates (simple vs. complex) and their impact is crucial for diabetes management.

- **Fiber Focus:** Choose complex carbohydrates rich in fiber, as fiber helps regulate blood sugar and promotes a feeling of fullness.

2. Protein's Role in Blood Sugar Stability:

- **Sustained Energy:** Including lean proteins in your diet helps stabilize blood sugar levels, as proteins are digested more slowly than carbohydrates.

- **Diverse Sources:** Diversify protein sources with lean meats, poultry, fish, tofu, legumes, and low-fat dairy.

3. Fats for Heart Health and Blood Sugar Control:

- **Healthy Fats:** Prioritize sources of monounsaturated and polyunsaturated fats, such as avocados, nuts, seeds, and olive oil, to support heart health and stabilize blood sugar.

- **Moderation is Key:** While fats are essential, be mindful of portion sizes to manage calorie intake.

Embracing a Balanced Plate:

4. Portion Control and Mindful Eating:

- **Quality over Quantity:** Focus on the quality of the foods you eat and practice mindful eating to prevent overconsumption.

- **Portion Awareness:** Use smaller plates, measure servings, and pay attention to portion sizes to avoid unnecessary calorie intake.

5. Incorporating a Variety of Nutrient-Dense Foods:

- **Colorful Plate:** Include a variety of colorful fruits, vegetables, whole grains, and lean proteins to ensure a broad range of nutrients.

- **Vitamins and Minerals:** These foods provide essential vitamins and minerals that contribute to overall health and support the body's ability to manage diabetes.

Practical Tips for Holistic Diabetes Management:

6. Hydration and Blood Sugar Regulation:

- **Importance of Water:** Stay hydrated with water, as it plays a role in digestion, nutrient absorption, and blood sugar regulation.

- **Limit Sugary Drinks:** Avoid sugary beverages that can cause rapid spikes in blood sugar.

7. Meal Timing and Consistency:

- **Consistent Schedule:** Maintain regular meal times to establish a routine that helps regulate blood sugar levels.

- **Balanced Snacks:** Plan for balanced snacks between meals to prevent extreme blood sugar fluctuations.

8. Individualized Approach with Professional Guidance:

- **Consult with Healthcare Professionals:** Collaborate with healthcare providers and nutritionists to create an individualized meal plan that considers specific health needs, preferences, and lifestyle.

- **Regular Monitoring and Adjustments:** Regularly monitor blood sugar levels and make adjustments to the meal plan as needed.

Holistic Lifestyle Integration:

9. Physical Activity and Well-Being:

   - **Exercise and Blood Sugar Control:** Integrate regular physical activity into your routine to improve insulin sensitivity and support overall well-being.

   - **Coordinate Meals and Exercise:** Time your meals and snacks to complement your exercise routine for optimal results.

10. Stress Management:

   - **Impact on Blood Sugar:** Recognize the connection between stress and blood sugar levels. Incorporate stress management techniques such as meditation, deep breathing, or yoga into your daily routine.

A holistic approach to diabetes management involves more than just monitoring blood sugar levels. By adopting a balanced, nutrient-dense meal plan, staying mindful of portion sizes, and integrating healthy lifestyle practices, individuals with diabetes can achieve better control over their condition. This holistic approach not only supports blood sugar management but also contributes to overall health and well-being. Always consult with healthcare professionals for personalized advice and guidance in crafting a comprehensive diabetes management plan.

Carbohydrate Counting and Blood Sugar Control

Effective diabetes management often revolves around understanding and managing carbohydrate intake. Carbohydrates directly influence blood sugar levels, making carbohydrate counting a valuable tool for individuals with diabetes. This approach empowers individuals to make informed choices about their diet, promoting better blood sugar control. Here's a guide to incorporating carbohydrate counting into your meal planning for effective diabetes management:

1. The Importance of Carbohydrate Counting:

   - **Blood Sugar Impact:** Carbohydrates are broken down into glucose, impacting blood sugar levels. Counting carbohydrates helps manage the quantity and quality of these influences.

- **Individual Variability:** Different individuals may respond differently to the same amount of carbohydrates. Personalized carbohydrate counting allows for precise adjustments based on individual responses.

2. Learn to Read Food Labels:

- **Total Carbohydrates vs. Net Carbohydrates:** Understand the difference between total carbohydrates and net carbohydrates. Net carbohydrates are calculated by subtracting fiber and sugar alcohols from the total carbohydrate content.
- **Serving Sizes:** Pay attention to serving sizes on food labels to accurately assess carbohydrate content.

3. Identify High and Low-Glycemic Foods:

- **Glycemic Index (GI):** Familiarize yourself with the glycemic index, which measures how quickly a food raises blood sugar levels. Low-GI foods cause a slower, more gradual increase.

- **Prioritize Low-GI Foods:** Opt for low-GI foods such as whole grains, legumes, and non-starchy vegetables to minimize rapid blood sugar spikes.

4. Planning Balanced Meals with Carbohydrate Counting:

- **Distribute Carbs Throughout the Day:** Instead of consuming a large amount of carbohydrates in one meal, distribute them evenly throughout the day to maintain stable blood sugar levels.

- **Combine with Proteins and Fats:** Pairing carbohydrates with proteins and healthy fats can help slow down digestion, moderating the impact on blood sugar.

5. Utilize Portion Control:

- **Measuring Tools:** Use measuring cups, a food scale, or visual references to gauge portion sizes accurately.

- **Mindful Eating:** Develop mindfulness around portion control to avoid overconsumption and maintain better blood sugar control.

6. Technology and Apps for Carbohydrate Tracking:

- **Mobile Apps:** Utilize mobile apps designed for tracking carbohydrates, which can simplify the process and provide valuable insights into daily intake.
- **Continuous Glucose Monitoring (CGM):** For those using CGM systems, integrate real-time data into your meal planning to observe the immediate impact of carbohydrate intake on blood sugar levels.

7. Professional Guidance and Education:

- **Dietitian Consultation:** Seek guidance from a registered dietitian to tailor carbohydrate counting to your individual needs and lifestyle.
- **Educational Resources:** Take advantage of educational materials and resources provided by

healthcare professionals to enhance your understanding of carbohydrate counting.

8. Regular Monitoring and Adjustments:

- **Blood Sugar Monitoring:** Regularly monitor blood sugar levels to assess the impact of different carbohydrate amounts and adjust your meal plan accordingly.

- **Consult with Healthcare Team:** Collaborate with your healthcare team to make informed decisions about medication adjustments based on carbohydrate counting and blood sugar patterns.

Carbohydrate counting is a powerful strategy for individuals with diabetes, offering a nuanced and personalized approach to meal planning. By understanding the impact of carbohydrates, reading food labels, utilizing portion control, and incorporating technology, individuals can gain better control over their blood sugar levels. Remember, this approach is most effective when combined with regular monitoring, professional guidance, and a holistic approach to diabetes management. Always consult with your healthcare team for personalized advice and adjustments to your meal plan.

Smart Snacking for Diabetes

Snacking plays a crucial role in diabetes management, providing an opportunity to maintain blood sugar levels and stave off hunger between meals. However, it's essential to approach snacking with mindfulness, choosing nutrient-dense options that contribute to overall health and help control blood sugar. Here's a guide to smart snacking for effective diabetes management:

1. Embrace Nutrient-Dense Snack Options:

- **Fresh Fruits and Vegetables:** Incorporate fresh fruits and vegetables into your snacks. These provide essential vitamins, minerals, and fiber while being low in calories.
- **Nuts and Seeds:** Opt for unsalted nuts and seeds, which offer healthy fats, protein, and fiber.

They contribute to a feeling of fullness and help stabilize blood sugar.

- **Greek Yogurt:** Choose plain, low-fat Greek yogurt for a protein-packed snack. Add berries or a drizzle of honey for sweetness without excessive sugar.

2. Mindful Carbohydrate Choices:

- **Whole Grains:** Select whole grains for a slow-release energy boost. Whole grain crackers, oatmeal, or whole grain bread with nut butter are excellent choices.
- **Legumes:** Incorporate legumes like chickpeas or hummus for a combination of protein and complex carbohydrates.

3. Portion Control is Key:

- **Pre-portioned Snacks:** Divide snacks into pre-portioned servings to avoid overeating. This helps manage calorie intake and keeps blood sugar levels in check.

- **Use Small Plates or Bowls:** Opt for smaller plates or bowls to create the illusion of a fuller portion.

4. Protein-Packed Options:

- **Cheese and Whole Grain Crackers:** Pairing a small serving of cheese with whole grain crackers provides a satisfying combination of protein and carbohydrates.
- **Hard-Boiled Eggs:** Hard-boiled eggs are a convenient, protein-rich snack that contributes to a sense of fullness.

5. Hydration and Snacking:

- **Water as a Snack:** Stay hydrated by choosing water as your primary beverage. Sometimes, feelings of hunger are actually signs of dehydration.
- **Infused Water:** Add a slice of lemon, cucumber, or berries to your water for a refreshing twist.

6. Plan Ahead for Success:

- **Prepared Snack Packs:** Prepare snack packs with a mix of nuts, seeds, and dried fruits. Having these readily available makes it easier to make healthy choices.

- **Vegetable Sticks and Hummus:** Pre-cut vegetable sticks paired with hummus make for a convenient and nutritious snack.

7. Avoid Highly Processed Snacks:

- **Read Labels:** Be vigilant about reading labels to identify added sugars and unhealthy fats in packaged snacks.

- **Opt for Whole Foods:** Choose whole, minimally processed foods over highly processed snacks to support overall health.

8. Timing Matters:

- **Snack Timing:** Plan snacks strategically between meals to prevent extreme fluctuations in blood sugar levels.

- **Pre-Exercise Snack:** If you're engaging in physical activity, have a small, balanced snack beforehand to maintain energy levels.

9. Continuous Glucose Monitoring (CGM) Integration:

- **Utilize Real-Time Data:** If using CGM, leverage real-time data to observe how different snacks affect your blood sugar levels. Adjust your snack choices based on this information.

Smart snacking is a valuable component of diabetes management, contributing to stable blood sugar levels and overall well-being. By choosing nutrient-dense options, practicing portion control, and planning ahead, individuals with diabetes can enjoy satisfying snacks without compromising their health goals. It's crucial to integrate smart snacking into a comprehensive meal plan, working in tandem with other aspects of diabetes management. As always, consult with your healthcare team for personalized advice and adjustments to your snacking routine.

Chapter 4: Delicious Pritikin Breakfast Recipes

The Pritikin Program is renowned for its focus on healthy living and promoting heart-healthy nutrition. Breakfast, being the most important meal of the day, plays a crucial role in starting your day on a nutritious note. Pritikin breakfast recipes not only prioritize health but also tantalize the taste buds with a variety of flavors. Here are some delicious Pritikin breakfast recipes to kickstart your day:

1. Oatmeal with Fresh Berries:

   - Ingredients:

   - 1/2 cup old-fashioned oats

   - 1 cup water

   - 1/2 cup mixed fresh berries (strawberries, blueberries, raspberries)

   - 1 tablespoon chopped nuts (almonds, walnuts)

   - 1/2 teaspoon cinnamon

- Instructions:

- Cook the oats with water according to package instructions.

- Top with fresh berries, chopped nuts, and a sprinkle of cinnamon.

2. Greek Yogurt Parfait:

- Ingredients:

- 1 cup non-fat Greek yogurt
- 1/2 cup granola (look for a low-sugar, whole-grain option)
- 1/2 cup sliced bananas
- 1 tablespoon honey

- Instructions:

- In a glass or bowl, layer Greek yogurt, granola, and sliced bananas.

- Drizzle with honey for a touch of sweetness.

3. Vegetable Omelette:

- Ingredients:

- 2 eggs
- 1/4 cup diced bell peppers
- 1/4 cup diced tomatoes

- 1/4 cup chopped spinach

- Salt and pepper to taste

- **Instructions:**

- Whisk eggs in a bowl and season with salt and pepper.

- In a non-stick pan, sauté bell peppers, tomatoes, and spinach until tender.

- Pour whisked eggs over the vegetables and cook until the omelette is set.

4. Whole Grain Toast with Avocado:

- **Ingredients:**

- 2 slices whole-grain bread

- 1/2 ripe avocado

- Salt, pepper, and red pepper flakes to taste

- **Instructions:**

- Toast the whole-grain bread slices.

- Mash the avocado and spread it over the toast.

- Sprinkle with salt, pepper, and red pepper flakes for added flavor.

5. Smoothie Bowl:

- Ingredients:

- 1 cup frozen mixed berries

- 1/2 banana

- 1/2 cup unsweetened almond milk

- 1 tablespoon chia seeds

- Toppings: sliced strawberries, granola, and a drizzle of honey

- Instructions:

- Blend frozen berries, banana, and almond milk until smooth.

- Pour the smoothie into a bowl and top with chia seeds, sliced strawberries, granola, and a drizzle of honey.

These Pritikin breakfast recipes provide a perfect balance of nutrients to fuel your day while adhering to the principles of a heart-healthy diet. Experiment with these recipes and feel free to customize them to suit your taste preferences and dietary needs. Enjoy a delicious and nutritious start to your mornings!

Energizing Breakfast Ideas

Starting your day with an energizing breakfast is key to maintaining vitality and focus throughout the morning. The Pritikin Program, known for its emphasis on heart-healthy living, offers a range of breakfast options that not only taste delightful but also provide the energy needed to kickstart your day. Here are some energizing Pritikin breakfast recipes to fuel your mornings:

1. Quinoa Breakfast Bowl:

- **Ingredients:**
- 1/2 cup cooked quinoa
- 1/4 cup diced mango
- 1/4 cup diced pineapple
- 1 tablespoon shredded coconut
- 1 tablespoon chopped nuts (such as almonds or pistachios)

- Instructions:

- Combine cooked quinoa with diced mango, pineapple, shredded coconut, and chopped nuts for a tropical and protein-packed breakfast.

2. Egg and Veggie Wrap:

-Ingredients:

- 2 egg whites
- 1 whole-grain wrap
- 1/4 cup diced bell peppers
- 1/4 cup spinach
- Salsa for topping

- Instructions:

- Scramble egg whites in a pan with diced bell peppers and spinach.

- Place the scrambled mixture in a whole-grain wrap, and top with salsa for a satisfying, protein-rich breakfast.

3. Chia Seed Pudding:

- Ingredients:

- 2 tablespoons chia seeds
- 1/2 cup unsweetened almond milk
- 1/2 teaspoon vanilla extract
- Fresh berries for topping

- Instructions:

- Mix chia seeds with almond milk and vanilla extract, then refrigerate overnight.

- Top with fresh berries in the morning for a nutrient-packed and energizing pudding.

4. Sweet Potato Breakfast Hash:

  - Ingredients:
  - 1 medium sweet potato, diced
  - 1/4 cup black beans (canned and rinsed)
  - 1/4 cup diced tomatoes
  - 1 teaspoon olive oil
  - 1/2 teaspoon cumin

  - Instructions:

- Sauté diced sweet potato in olive oil until golden brown, then add black beans, diced tomatoes, and cumin for a savory and energizing breakfast hash.

5. Protein-Packed Smoothie:

  - Ingredients:
  - 1 cup spinach
  - 1/2 banana
  - 1/2 cup Greek yogurt

- 1 tablespoon almond butter

- 1/2 cup water or unsweetened almond milk

- Instructions:

- Blend spinach, banana, Greek yogurt, almond butter, and water/almond milk for a refreshing and protein-rich smoothie to start your day.

These Pritikin breakfast recipes not only provide a burst of energy but also deliver essential nutrients to support overall well-being. Feel free to customize these recipes based on your preferences, and enjoy the benefits of a delicious and energizing breakfast that sets a positive tone for the rest of your day.

Morning Smoothies and Juices

Embracing a health-focused lifestyle often begins with the first meal of the day. Pritikin breakfast recipes are designed to provide a nutritious and delicious start to your mornings. Incorporating morning smoothies and juices into your breakfast routine can be an excellent way to kickstart your day with a burst of flavor and essential nutrients. Here are some delightful Pritikin recipes for morning smoothies and juices:

1. Green Goodness Smoothie:

- Ingredients:

  - 1 cup kale or spinach
  - 1/2 cucumber, peeled and sliced
  - 1/2 green apple, cored
  - 1/2 lemon, juiced
  - 1/2 cup water or coconut water
  - Ice cubes

- Instructions:

  - Blend kale/spinach, cucumber, green apple, lemon juice, and water until smooth.
  - Add ice cubes and blend again for a refreshing green smoothie.

2. Berry Blast Smoothie:

- Ingredients:

  - 1/2 cup strawberries
  - 1/2 cup blueberries
  - 1/2 cup raspberries

- 1/2 banana

- 1 cup unsweetened almond milk

- 1 tablespoon chia seeds

- Instructions:

- Blend strawberries, blueberries, raspberries, banana, and almond milk until creamy.

- Stir in chia seeds for added texture and nutritional benefits.

3. Citrus Sunrise Juice:

- Ingredients:

- 2 oranges, peeled and segmented

- 1 grapefruit, peeled and segmented

- 1/2 lime, juiced

- 1 tablespoon fresh mint leaves

- Ice cubes

- Instructions:

- Juice the oranges and grapefruit, then mix in lime juice.

- Pour over ice and garnish with fresh mint for a citrusy, invigorating morning juice.

4. Tropical Paradise Smoothie:

  - Ingredients:

   - 1/2 cup pineapple chunks

   - 1/2 mango, peeled and diced

   - 1/2 banana

   - 1/2 cup coconut water

   - 1 tablespoon flaxseeds

  - Instructions:

   - Blend pineapple, mango, banana, and coconut water until smooth.

   - Add flaxseeds for a dose of omega-3 fatty acids.

5. Carrot-Orange Energizer Juice:

  - Ingredients:

   - 2 carrots, peeled and chopped

   - 2 oranges, peeled and segmented

   - 1-inch piece of ginger, peeled

   - 1/2 cup water

   - Ice cubes

  - Instructions:

   - Juice carrots, oranges, and ginger.

- Dilute with water, pour over ice, and enjoy a zesty carrot-orange energizer.

These Pritikin morning smoothies and juices are not only delicious but also packed with vitamins, minerals, and antioxidants to jumpstart your day with a healthy dose of energy. Feel free to experiment with different combinations and tailor these recipes to suit your taste preferences and nutritional needs. Cheers to a vibrant and nutritious start!

Hearty Whole-Grain Breakfasts

A hearty and wholesome breakfast is a cornerstone of the Pritikin Program, emphasizing the importance of whole grains for sustained energy and overall health. These delicious Pritikin breakfast recipes showcase the goodness of whole grains, offering a variety of options to keep you satisfied throughout the morning. Dive into these hearty whole-grain breakfast ideas:

1. Quinoa and Fruit Breakfast Bowl:

- Ingredients:

- 1/2 cup cooked quinoa

- 1/2 cup mixed berries (strawberries, blueberries, raspberries)

- 1/4 cup chopped nuts (walnuts, almonds)

- 1 tablespoon honey or maple syrup

- Instructions:

- Combine cooked quinoa with mixed berries and top with chopped nuts.

- Drizzle with honey or maple syrup for a sweet and protein-packed bowl.

2. Whole Grain Pancakes:

- Ingredients:

- 1 cup whole wheat flour

- 1 tablespoon baking powder

- 1 tablespoon honey

- 1 cup almond milk

- Fresh fruit for topping

- Instructions:

- Mix whole wheat flour, baking powder, honey, and almond milk to form a batter.

- Cook pancakes on a non-stick pan and serve with your favorite fresh fruit.

3. Steel-Cut Oatmeal with Nut Butter:

- Ingredients:

- 1/2 cup steel-cut oats
- 1 1/2 cups water
- 1 tablespoon almond or peanut butter
- 1/2 banana, sliced

- Instructions:

- Cook steel-cut oats with water until creamy.

- Stir in nut butter and top with banana slices for a comforting and protein-rich breakfast.

4. Whole Grain Breakfast Burrito:

- Ingredients:

- 1 whole-grain tortilla
- 2 eggs, scrambled
- 1/4 cup black beans (canned and rinsed)
- Salsa and avocado for topping

- Instructions:

- Fill a whole-grain tortilla with scrambled eggs, black beans, salsa, and sliced avocado for a savory and filling breakfast burrito.

5. Brown Rice Pudding:

- Ingredients:

- 1 cup cooked brown rice
- 1 1/2 cups unsweetened almond milk
- 1 teaspoon vanilla extract
- Cinnamon and raisins for garnish

- Instructions:

- Simmer cooked brown rice with almond milk and vanilla extract until creamy.
- Sprinkle with cinnamon and garnish with raisins for a warm and satisfying rice pudding.

These Pritikin whole-grain breakfast recipes provide a hearty foundation for your day, combining the goodness of whole grains with flavorful ingredients. Experiment with these recipes, and feel free to customize them to suit your taste preferences while enjoying the benefits of a nourishing and heart-healthy breakfast.

Creative Oatmeal and Cereal Options

Oatmeal and cereals take center stage in the Pritikin breakfast repertoire, offering a canvas for creativity and nutrition. These recipes not only elevate the humble oatmeal and cereal but also provide a nutritious and delicious start to your day. Explore the following creative Pritikin breakfast ideas:

1. Pumpkin Spice Oatmeal:
  - **Ingredients:**
    - 1/2 cup old-fashioned oats
    - 1 cup water
    - 1/4 cup canned pumpkin puree
    - 1/2 teaspoon pumpkin spice
    - Chopped pecans for topping

  - **Instructions:**

- Cook oats with water and stir in pumpkin puree and pumpkin spice.

- Top with chopped pecans for a warm and comforting fall-inspired breakfast.

2. Coconut Chia Seed Pudding:

- **Ingredients:**

  - 2 tablespoons chia seeds
  - 1/2 cup unsweetened coconut milk
  - 1/2 teaspoon vanilla extract
  - Sliced kiwi and toasted coconut for garnish

- **Instructions:**

- Mix chia seeds with coconut milk and vanilla extract, then refrigerate overnight.

- Garnish with sliced kiwi and toasted coconut for a tropical twist.

3. Blueberry Almond Crunch Cereal Bowl:

- **Ingredients:**

  - 1 cup whole grain cereal
  - 1/2 cup fresh blueberries
  - 1 tablespoon almond butter
  - Unsweetened almond milk

- Instructions:

- Combine whole grain cereal with fresh blueberries.

- Drizzle with almond butter and pour almond milk for a crunchy and satisfying breakfast.

4. Apple Cinnamon Quinoa Bowl:

- Ingredients:

- 1/2 cup cooked quinoa

- 1/2 apple, diced

- 1/2 teaspoon cinnamon

- 1 tablespoon chopped walnuts

- Instructions:

- Mix cooked quinoa with diced apple and sprinkle with cinnamon.

- Top with chopped walnuts for a wholesome and flavorful quinoa bowl.

5. Tropical Granola Parfait:

- Ingredients:

- 1/2 cup low-sugar granola

- 1/2 cup Greek yogurt

- 1/4 cup diced pineapple

- 1/4 cup mango chunks

- **Instructions:**

- Layer granola, Greek yogurt, diced pineapple, and mango for a tropical and satisfying parfait.

These Pritikin oatmeal and cereal options provide a perfect blend of creativity and nutrition, ensuring a delicious and wholesome start to your day. Tailor these recipes to your taste preferences and relish the variety of flavors and textures that make breakfast a delightful experience while maintaining a commitment to a heart-healthy lifestyle.

Chapter 5: Wholesome Lunch and Dinner Recipes

Certainly! Wholesome lunch and dinner recipes are not only delicious but also provide essential nutrients to fuel your body throughout the day. Here are some nutritious and flavorful recipes that you can enjoy for lunch or dinner:

1. Quinoa Salad Bowl:

Ingredients:

- 1 cup quinoa, cooked

- 1 cup cherry tomatoes, halved

- 1 cucumber, diced

- 1 bell pepper, chopped

- 1/2 red onion, finely chopped

- 1/4 cup feta cheese, crumbled

- 2 tablespoons olive oil

- 1 tablespoon balsamic vinegar

- Salt and pepper to taste

Instructions:

1. In a large bowl, combine the cooked quinoa, cherry tomatoes, cucumber, bell pepper, and red onion.

2. In a small bowl, whisk together the olive oil and balsamic vinegar. Pour the dressing over the salad and toss to combine.

3. Sprinkle feta cheese on top and season with salt and pepper.

4. Serve chilled and enjoy a protein-packed, nutrient-rich meal.

2. Grilled Chicken with Roasted Vegetables:

Ingredients:

- 4 boneless, skinless chicken breasts
- 2 tablespoons olive oil
- 1 teaspoon garlic powder
- 1 teaspoon dried oregano
- 1 teaspoon paprika
- Salt and pepper to taste
- Assorted vegetables (carrots, broccoli, bell peppers)

Instructions:

1. Preheat the grill or grill pan.

2. In a bowl, mix olive oil, garlic powder, oregano, paprika, salt, and pepper to create a marinade.

3. Coat chicken breasts with the marinade and let them sit for at least 30 minutes.

4. Grill the chicken until fully cooked, about 6-8 minutes per side.

5. In a separate baking sheet, toss assorted vegetables with olive oil, salt, and pepper. Roast in the oven at 400°F (200°C) for 20-25 minutes.

6. Serve the grilled chicken over a bed of roasted vegetables for a well-balanced and satisfying meal.

3. Vegetarian Stir-Fry:

Ingredients:

- 1 cup tofu, cubed

- 2 cups broccoli florets

- 1 bell pepper, sliced

- 1 carrot, julienned

- 1 cup snap peas

- 3 tablespoons soy sauce

- 1 tablespoon sesame oil

- 2 cloves garlic, minced

- 1 teaspoon ginger, grated

- Cooked brown rice

Instructions:

1. In a wok or large pan, heat sesame oil over medium-high heat.

2. Add tofu and stir-fry until golden brown. Remove from the pan and set aside.

3. In the same pan, add a bit more oil if needed. Stir-fry garlic and ginger until fragrant.

4. Add broccoli, bell pepper, carrot, and snap peas. Cook until vegetables are tender-crisp.

5. Return the tofu to the pan, add soy sauce, and toss everything together.

6. Serve the stir-fry over cooked brown rice for a quick and nutritious vegetarian dinner.

These recipes offer a variety of flavors while ensuring you get a well-rounded mix of nutrients for a wholesome lunch or dinner. Adjust ingredients to suit your taste preferences and dietary needs. Enjoy your nutritious and delicious meals!

Satisfying Salads and Dressings

Satisfying salads are a fantastic option for wholesome lunches and dinners, providing a mix of textures, flavors, and nutrients. Pairing them with delicious homemade dressings elevates the dining experience. Here are some delightful salad recipes along with accompanying dressings:

1. Mango Avocado Chicken Salad:
Salad Ingredients:
- 2 cups mixed greens
- 1 cup grilled chicken, sliced
- 1 ripe mango, diced
- 1 avocado, sliced
- 1/4 cup red onion, thinly sliced
- 1/4 cup chopped cilantro
- 1/4 cup toasted almonds

Dressing:
- 2 tablespoons olive oil
- 1 tablespoon balsamic vinegar
- 1 teaspoon honey

- Salt and pepper to taste

Instructions:

1. In a large bowl, combine mixed greens, grilled chicken, mango, avocado, red onion, cilantro, and toasted almonds.

2. In a small bowl, whisk together olive oil, balsamic vinegar, honey, salt, and pepper to create the dressing.

3. Drizzle the dressing over the salad and toss gently to coat.

4. Serve immediately for a refreshing and satisfying meal.

2. Quinoa and Chickpea Power Salad:

Salad Ingredients:

- 1 cup cooked quinoa

- 1 can chickpeas, drained and rinsed

- 1 cup cherry tomatoes, halved

- 1 cucumber, diced

- 1/2 cup feta cheese, crumbled

- 1/4 cup Kalamata olives, sliced

- Fresh basil leaves, for garnish

Dressing:

- 3 tablespoons olive oil

- 1 tablespoon lemon juice

- 1 teaspoon Dijon mustard

- 1 clove garlic, minced

- Salt and pepper to taste

Instructions:

1. In a large bowl, combine quinoa, chickpeas, cherry tomatoes, cucumber, feta cheese, and Kalamata olives.

2. In a small bowl, whisk together olive oil, lemon juice, Dijon mustard, garlic, salt, and pepper to make the dressing.

3. Pour the dressing over the salad and toss gently to combine.

4. Garnish with fresh basil leaves and serve this protein-packed salad.

3. Caprese Salad with Balsamic Glaze:

Salad Ingredients:

- 2 cups cherry tomatoes, halved

- 1 cup fresh mozzarella balls

- Fresh basil leaves

- Salt and pepper to taste
- Balsamic glaze for drizzling

Dressing:
- 3 tablespoons extra-virgin olive oil
- 2 tablespoons balsamic vinegar
- 1 teaspoon honey
- 1 teaspoon Dijon mustard

Instructions:
1. Arrange cherry tomatoes and fresh mozzarella on a serving platter. Tuck fresh basil leaves in between.
2. In a small bowl, whisk together olive oil, balsamic vinegar, honey, and Dijon mustard for the dressing.
3. Drizzle the dressing over the salad, season with salt and pepper, and finish with a generous drizzle of balsamic glaze.
4. Serve this classic Caprese salad as a light and flavorful lunch or dinner.

These salad recipes are not only nutritious but also bursting with vibrant colors and flavors. The homemade dressings add a personal touch and enhance the overall dining experience. Enjoy these wholesome salads as a satisfying and healthful meal option.

Flavorful Vegetable-Based Dishes

Vegetable-based dishes are not only nutritious but also bursting with flavor. Incorporating a variety of vegetables into your lunch and dinner can create satisfying and wholesome meals. Here are some flavorful vegetable-based recipes to try:

1. Roasted Vegetable and Chickpea Buddha Bowl:

Ingredients:
- 1 sweet potato, cubed
- 1 zucchini, sliced
- 1 red bell pepper, chopped
- 1 cup cherry tomatoes
- 1 can chickpeas, drained and rinsed
- 2 tablespoons olive oil
- 1 teaspoon cumin

- 1 teaspoon paprika

- Salt and pepper to taste

- Quinoa or brown rice (for serving)

Instructions:

1. Preheat the oven to 400°F (200°C).

2. In a large bowl, toss sweet potato, zucchini, red bell pepper, cherry tomatoes, and chickpeas with olive oil, cumin, paprika, salt, and pepper.

3. Spread the vegetables and chickpeas on a baking sheet and roast for 25-30 minutes or until golden and crispy.

4. Serve the roasted vegetables and chickpeas over a bed of quinoa or brown rice for a delicious and filling Buddha bowl.

2. Eggplant and Tomato Ratatouille:

Ingredients:

- 1 large eggplant, diced

- 2 zucchinis, sliced

- 1 bell pepper, diced

- 1 onion, chopped

- 3 cloves garlic, minced

- 1 can diced tomatoes

- 2 tablespoons tomato paste

- 1 teaspoon dried thyme

- 1 teaspoon dried rosemary

- Salt and pepper to taste

Instructions:

1. In a large pot, sauté onion and garlic until softened.

2. Add eggplant, zucchini, bell pepper, diced tomatoes, tomato paste, thyme, rosemary, salt, and pepper.

3. Simmer on low heat for 30-40 minutes, stirring occasionally until the vegetables are tender.

4. Serve the ratatouille on its own or over whole grain pasta for a hearty and flavorful dinner.

3. Stir-Fried Tofu and Vegetable Noodles:

Ingredients:

- 8 oz (225g) rice noodles

- 1 block extra-firm tofu, pressed and cubed

- 2 tablespoons soy sauce

- 1 tablespoon sesame oil

- 1 tablespoon hoisin sauce

- 1 tablespoon vegetable oil

- 1 bell pepper, thinly sliced

- 1 carrot, julienned

- 1 cup broccoli florets

- 2 green onions, sliced

Instructions:

1. Cook rice noodles according to package instructions. Drain and set aside.

2. In a bowl, marinate tofu in soy sauce, sesame oil, and hoisin sauce.

3. Heat vegetable oil in a large pan or wok. Add tofu and stir-fry until golden.

4. Add bell pepper, carrot, and broccoli. Stir-fry until vegetables are tender-crisp.

5. Toss in the cooked noodles and green onions. Mix everything well.

6. Serve this flavorful stir-fry as a satisfying and quick vegetable-based dinner option.

These vegetable-based dishes are not only packed with nutrients but also deliver a burst of flavors to make your lunch and dinner both enjoyable and wholesome. Feel free to customize these recipes with your favorite veggies and spices.

Protein-Packed Plant-Based Entrees

Absolutely! Plant-based meals can be incredibly satisfying and protein-packed. Here are some delicious and nutritious lunch and dinner recipes featuring plant-based protein sources:

1. Chickpea and Spinach Coconut Curry:
Ingredients:
- 1 can chickpeas, drained and rinsed
- 2 cups spinach, chopped
- 1 can coconut milk
- 1 onion, diced
- 3 cloves garlic, minced
- 1 tablespoon curry powder
- 1 teaspoon turmeric
- Salt and pepper to taste
- Cooked quinoa or brown rice (for serving)

Instructions:

1. In a large pan, sauté onion and garlic until softened.

2. Add chickpeas, spinach, coconut milk, curry powder, turmeric, salt, and pepper.

3. Simmer for 15-20 minutes until flavors meld and the spinach wilts.

4. Serve the curry over quinoa or brown rice for a protein-packed and flavorful plant-based entree.

2. Lentil and Vegetable Stuffed Peppers:

Ingredients:

- 4 bell peppers, halved and seeds removed
- 1 cup dry green or brown lentils, cooked
- 1 zucchini, diced
- 1 carrot, grated
- 1 cup diced tomatoes
- 1 onion, finely chopped
- 2 cloves garlic, minced
- 1 teaspoon cumin
- 1 teaspoon smoked paprika
- Salt and pepper to taste
- Vegan cheese (optional, for topping)

Instructions:

1. Preheat the oven to 375°F (190°C).

2. In a pan, sauté onion and garlic until translucent. Add zucchini, carrot, diced tomatoes, cumin, smoked paprika, salt, and pepper.

3. Stir in cooked lentils and let the mixture simmer for 10 minutes.

4. Stuff the halved bell peppers with the lentil and vegetable mixture.

5. Bake for 25-30 minutes or until the peppers are tender.

6. Optionally, sprinkle vegan cheese on top during the last 5 minutes of baking.

7. Serve these stuffed peppers with a side salad for a wholesome and protein-rich meal.

3. Quinoa and Black Bean Enchilada Casserole:

Ingredients:

- 1 cup quinoa, cooked

- 1 can black beans, drained and rinsed

- 1 cup corn kernels (fresh or frozen)

- 1 bell pepper, diced

- 1 cup enchilada sauce

- 1 teaspoon cumin

- 1 teaspoon chili powder

- Salt and pepper to taste

- Avocado and cilantro for topping

Instructions:

1. Preheat the oven to 375°F (190°C).

2. In a large bowl, mix quinoa, black beans, corn, bell pepper, enchilada sauce, cumin, chili powder, salt, and pepper.

3. Transfer the mixture to a baking dish and spread it evenly.

4. Bake for 20-25 minutes until the casserole is heated through.

5. Top with sliced avocado and fresh cilantro before serving.

6. Enjoy this protein-packed, plant-based enchilada casserole as a satisfying dinner.

These recipes showcase that plant-based meals can be both protein-rich and full of flavor. Feel free to customize these recipes based on your preferences and dietary needs.

Savory Soups and Stews

Certainly! Soups and stews are not only comforting but also versatile and nutritious. They can be packed with a variety of vegetables, legumes, and grains to create wholesome and satisfying meals. Here are some savory soup and stew recipes for wholesome lunches and dinners:

1. Minestrone Soup:

Ingredients:

- 1 tablespoon olive oil

- 1 onion, diced

- 2 carrots, sliced

- 2 celery stalks, chopped

- 3 cloves garlic, minced

- 1 can (15 oz) kidney beans, drained and rinsed

- 1 can (15 oz) diced tomatoes

- 1 zucchini, diced

- 1 cup green beans, chopped

- 1 cup small pasta (e.g., ditalini or elbow)

- 6 cups vegetable broth

- 1 teaspoon dried oregano

- 1 teaspoon dried basil

- Salt and pepper to taste

- Fresh parsley for garnish

Instructions:

1. In a large pot, heat olive oil over medium heat. Sauté onion, carrots, celery, and garlic until softened.

2. Add kidney beans, diced tomatoes, zucchini, green beans, pasta, vegetable broth, oregano, basil, salt, and pepper.

3. Simmer for 20-25 minutes or until the vegetables and pasta are tender.

4. Garnish with fresh parsley before serving. Enjoy this hearty and flavorful minestrone soup.

2. Sweet Potato and Black Bean Chili:

Ingredients:

- 2 sweet potatoes, peeled and diced

- 1 can (15 oz) black beans, drained and rinsed

- 1 can (15 oz) diced tomatoes

- 1 onion, diced

- 3 cloves garlic, minced

- 1 bell pepper, diced

- 1 tablespoon chili powder

- 1 teaspoon cumin

- 1/2 teaspoon smoked paprika
- 4 cups vegetable broth
- Salt and pepper to taste
- Avocado and cilantro for topping

Instructions:

1. In a large pot, combine sweet potatoes, black beans, diced tomatoes, onion, garlic, bell pepper, chili powder, cumin, smoked paprika, vegetable broth, salt, and pepper.

2. Bring to a boil, then reduce heat and simmer for 20-25 minutes or until sweet potatoes are tender.

3. Serve the chili topped with sliced avocado and fresh cilantro for a protein-packed and satisfying dinner.

3. Lentil and Kale Stew:

Ingredients:

- 1 cup dry green or brown lentils, rinsed
- 1 onion, diced
- 3 carrots, sliced
- 3 celery stalks, chopped
- 3 cloves garlic, minced
- 1 can (15 oz) diced tomatoes

- 1 bunch kale, stems removed and leaves chopped
- 6 cups vegetable broth
- 1 teaspoon dried thyme
- 1 teaspoon smoked paprika
- Salt and pepper to taste

Instructions:

1. In a large pot, combine lentils, onion, carrots, celery, garlic, diced tomatoes, kale, vegetable broth, thyme, smoked paprika, salt, and pepper.
2. Bring to a boil, then reduce heat and simmer for 25-30 minutes or until lentils are tender.
3. Adjust seasoning as needed and serve this hearty lentil and kale stew for a wholesome and nutritious meal.

These savory soup and stew recipes are not only delicious but also filled with nourishing ingredients. Feel free to customize the recipes based on your preferences and enjoy a warm and satisfying lunch or dinner.

Chapter 6: Sweet and Healthy Desserts

In a world where health-conscious choices are becoming increasingly prevalent, the notion of indulging in sweet treats need not be synonymous with compromising one's well-being. The realm of desserts has evolved, offering a plethora of options that marry the realms of deliciousness and nutrition. Discover the delightful universe of sweet and healthy desserts that not only satisfy your sweet tooth but also contribute to your overall well-being.

1. Fruit Infusions: Nature's Candy

Embrace the vibrant and natural sweetness of fruits to create desserts that are not only delicious but also packed with essential vitamins and minerals. Whether it's a refreshing fruit salad, a berry parfait, or grilled pineapple skewers, incorporating fresh fruits into your desserts adds a burst of flavors without the need for excessive sugar.

2. Wholesome Baking: Flour Alternatives and Nut Butters

Traditional baking often relies on refined flours and sugars. Explore the world of wholesome baking by incorporating alternative flours like almond flour, coconut flour, or oat flour. These alternatives not only impart a unique flavor but also bring added nutritional benefits. Nut butters, such as almond or cashew butter, can replace traditional fats, adding a creamy texture and a dose of healthy fats to your desserts.

3. Yogurt Delights: Creaminess without Guilt

Yogurt is a versatile ingredient that can be transformed into a variety of sweet treats. Opt for Greek yogurt for a protein boost, and pair it with honey, fresh fruits, or a drizzle of dark chocolate for a guilt-free dessert. Frozen yogurt popsicles, yogurt parfaits, and yogurt-based smoothie bowls are just a few examples of how this dairy delight can be incorporated into your sweet repertoire.

4. Date-Sweetened Goodies: Nature's Caramel

Dates are a natural sweetener that can elevate your desserts without the need for refined sugars. Whether blended into a date paste for baking or simply stuffed with nuts, these chewy delights bring a rich, caramel-like sweetness to your treats. Try date and nut energy balls, date-stuffed oat bars, or date-sweetened puddings for a healthy twist on classic desserts.

5. Dark Chocolate Elegance: Decadence with Benefits

Dark chocolate is not only a decadent treat but also offers health benefits. Rich in antioxidants and lower in sugar than milk chocolate, dark chocolate can be melted and drizzled over fruit, used as a dip for nuts, or incorporated into energy bites. Experiment with different cocoa percentages to find your preferred balance of sweetness and intensity.

Indulging in sweet and healthy desserts is not just a treat for your taste buds but also a commitment to your well-being. By exploring natural sweeteners, alternative flours, and nutrient-dense ingredients, you can create a dessert repertoire that satisfies your cravings without compromising your health goals. So, go ahead and enjoy the sweet side of life guilt-free!

Mindful Dessert Choices

In a world where mindful living is gaining prominence, the choices we make extend beyond our daily routines to include our dietary decisions. Desserts, often associated with indulgence and guilty pleasures, are not exempt from this shift toward conscious consumption. Embracing sweet and healthy desserts allows us to satisfy our cravings while maintaining a mindful approach to overall well-being.

1. Mindful Ingredient Selection: Nourishment in Every Bite

The foundation of a sweet and healthy dessert begins with mindful ingredient selection. Opt for wholesome, unprocessed components such as whole grains, nuts, seeds, and fresh fruits. By choosing nutrient-dense ingredients, you not only enhance the flavor profile but also infuse your desserts with essential vitamins, minerals, and antioxidants.

2. Balancing Sweetness: Natural Sweeteners and Moderation

Mindful dessert choices involve reimagining sweetness. Explore the spectrum of natural sweeteners like honey, maple syrup, or agave nectar, which provide a delightful sweetness without the drawbacks of refined sugars. Embrace moderation, savoring the natural flavors of ingredients rather than overwhelming your palate with excessive sweetness. This approach not only supports your health goals but also cultivates a deeper appreciation for the subtleties of taste.

3. Texture Harmony: Crispy, Creamy, and Chewy Delights

Mindful indulgence extends beyond taste to encompass the diverse textures that desserts offer. Create a harmonious blend of textures by incorporating elements such as crunchy nuts, creamy yogurts, or chewy dried fruits. The interplay of textures not only enhances the sensory experience but also fosters a more mindful and enjoyable dessert consumption.

4. Portion Control: Savoring Every Mouthful

In a world of supersized portions, practicing portion control is a mindful choice that promotes a healthier relationship with food. Whether it's a petite serving of a decadent chocolate mousse or a modest slice of a fruit-infused cake, savoring smaller portions allows you to fully enjoy the flavors without overindulging.

5. Creative Presentation: Elevating the Experience

Mindful dessert choices extend to the presentation, transforming the act of indulgence into an artful experience. Experiment with creative plating, garnishes, and serving methods to elevate the visual appeal of your sweet creations. A beautifully presented dessert not only enhances the dining experience but also encourages a more mindful and intentional approach to consumption.

Sweet and healthy desserts need not be a compromise; rather, they can be a celebration of mindful choices that honor both your taste buds and your well-being. By embracing natural ingredients, balancing sweetness, considering textures, practicing portion control, and presenting your creations with flair, you can embark on a journey of mindful indulgence, savoring each sweet moment without losing sight of your health and wellness goals.

Fruit-Centric Dessert Delights

Nature's candy comes in the form of succulent fruits, offering a spectrum of flavors that can transform any dessert into a delightful and health-conscious treat. Explore the world of fruit-centric desserts that not only satisfy your sweet cravings but also infuse your palate with the goodness of vitamins, fiber, and natural sweetness.

1. Fresh Fruit Parfaits: Layers of Flavor and Nutrition

Elevate your dessert experience with a colorful array of fresh fruit parfaits. Alternate layers of ripe berries, sliced kiwi, and chunks of pineapple with creamy Greek yogurt or cottage cheese. Top it off with a sprinkle of granola or a drizzle of honey for added texture and sweetness. The result is a visually appealing and nutrient-packed dessert that caters to your sweet tooth while providing a wholesome treat.

2. Grilled Fruit Delicacies: Caramelized Goodness

Bring out the natural sweetness of fruits by grilling them to perfection. Whether it's peaches, pineapples, or watermelon, the caramelization on the grill enhances their flavors, creating a delectable dessert option. Serve grilled fruit slices with a dollop of Greek yogurt or a scoop of vanilla frozen yogurt for a simple yet indulgent treat.

3. Fruit Salsas and Compotes: A Burst of Freshness

Transform fruits into vibrant salsas or compotes that can be used as toppings, dips, or accompaniments. Combine diced mangoes, strawberries, and mint for a refreshing salsa, or simmer a medley of berries with a touch of honey to create a versatile compote. These fruit-based additions add a burst of freshness and complexity to desserts like yogurt bowls, pancakes, or whole-grain waffles.

4. Frozen Fruit Popsicles: Cool and Nourishing Treats

Beat the heat with homemade frozen fruit popsicles. Blend together a mixture of your favorite fruits—such as berries, citrus, and melons—add a splash of coconut water or yogurt, and freeze in popsicle molds. These frozen delights not only satisfy your sweet tooth but also provide a hydrating and vitamin-packed alternative to traditional sugary popsicles.

5. Fruit-Stuffed Dark Chocolate: A Decadent Fusion

Combine the richness of dark chocolate with the freshness of fruit by creating fruit-stuffed chocolates. Dip strawberries, blueberries, or dried apricots in melted dark chocolate and let them set. The result is a decadent yet guilt-free treat that marries the antioxidant benefits of dark chocolate with the vitamins and minerals found in the fruit.

Fruit-centric desserts offer a vibrant and nutritious alternative to traditional sweet treats. By celebrating the natural sweetness and diversity of fruits, you can create desserts that not only satisfy your sweet cravings but also contribute to your overall well-being. Embrace the goodness of nature's bounty and treat yourself to a symphony of flavors with these delicious and healthy fruit-centric delights.

Nut and Seed–Based Sweet Treats

Dive into a world of wholesome indulgence with desserts that celebrate the nutritional powerhouse of nuts and seeds. Beyond their rich flavors and satisfying textures, nuts and seeds offer a treasure trove of essential nutrients. Explore a range of creative, nut and seed-based sweet treats that not only satiate your sweet cravings but also contribute to your overall well-being.

1. Nut Butter Bliss: Creamy Goodness in Every Bite

Nut butters, whether derived from almonds, peanuts, or cashews, are a versatile foundation for creating delicious and healthy desserts. Whip up no-bake energy bites by combining nut butter with oats, honey, and dark chocolate chips. Alternatively, use nut butter as a base for a guilt-free chocolate spread or drizzle it over fruit for a decadent touch that's high in healthy fats and protein.

2. Seeds of Sweetness: Chia Puddings and Flaxseed Bliss

Chia seeds and flaxseeds are small powerhouses of nutrition, packed with omega-3 fatty acids, fiber, and antioxidants. Create a delightful chia seed pudding by combining chia seeds with almond milk and letting it set. Layer it with fresh fruits or a dollop of Greek yogurt for a satisfying dessert that's as visually appealing as it is nutritious. Experiment with incorporating ground flaxseeds into baking for an extra boost of fiber and nutty flavor.

3. Nutty Crusts and Granola Parfaits: Crunchy Goodness

Replace traditional pastry crusts with nut-based alternatives to create healthier versions of pies and tarts. Almond flour or crushed nuts can form the foundation for a delectable crust that adds a satisfying crunch. Layer these crusts with Greek yogurt, fresh berries, and a sprinkle of homemade granola for a parfait that's not only delightful but also nutrient-dense.

4. Mixed Nut and Seed Bars: On-the-Go Nutrition

Craft your own nut and seed bars using a variety of nuts, seeds, and dried fruits. Blend together ingredients like almonds, walnuts, sunflower seeds, and chia seeds, binding them with natural sweeteners like honey or maple syrup. Press the mixture into bars and refrigerate until firm. These homemade bars offer a convenient, on-the-go option packed with protein, healthy fats, and fiber.

5. Nutty Frozen Delights: Ice Cream Alternatives

Experience the richness of frozen desserts without the guilt by experimenting with nut and seed-based alternatives. Create dairy-free ice cream using a base of blended cashews or almonds, sweetened with natural sweeteners and flavored with ingredients like vanilla, cocoa, or fruit. These frozen delights not only satisfy your sweet tooth but also provide a nutrient-rich alternative to traditional ice creams.

Nut and seed-based sweet treats open up a realm of possibilities for delicious, nutrient-packed desserts. By incorporating the goodness of nuts and seeds into your culinary creations, you not only enhance the flavor and texture but also infuse your desserts with essential nutrients. Embrace these wholesome alternatives to traditional sweets, and embark on a journey of sweet indulgence that nourishes both your taste buds and your well-being.

Baking Without Refined Sugar

In the quest for healthier dessert options, one of the most impactful choices is eliminating refined sugar from your baking repertoire. Discover the art of creating sweet and healthy desserts without compromising on taste by exploring alternative sweeteners and innovative baking techniques. From guilt-free cookies to wholesome cakes, embark on a journey to master the craft of baking without refined sugar.

1. Natural Sweeteners: A Symphony of Flavors

Replace refined sugar with a variety of natural sweeteners to add depth and nuance to your desserts. Experiment with honey, maple syrup, agave nectar, or date paste as alternatives. Each sweetener brings its unique flavor profile, allowing you to tailor your desserts to your taste preferences. Harness the natural sweetness of these alternatives while benefitting from additional nutrients and antioxidants.

2. Fruit Purees and Mashes: Nature's Sweet Bounty

Utilize the natural sugars found in fruits to sweeten your baked goods. Purees and mashes from fruits like bananas, apples, or sweet potatoes not only add sweetness but also contribute moisture to your recipes. Banana bread, applesauce muffins, and sweet potato brownies are just a few examples of how these fruit-based alternatives can elevate your baked treats.

3. Whole Grain Flours: Nutrient-Rich Foundations

Swap out refined flours for whole grain alternatives like whole wheat, oat, or almond flour. Whole grain flours not only impart a nuttier flavor and heartier texture but also bring a host of additional nutrients, including fiber and vitamins. Experiment with different flour combinations to achieve the desired texture while boosting the nutritional value of your desserts.

4. Dried Fruits and Nuts: Texture and Natural Sweetness

Introduce natural sweetness and textural elements to your desserts by incorporating dried fruits and nuts. Chopped dates, raisins, or dried figs not only add a burst of natural sweetness but also contribute chewiness and depth to your recipes. Nuts, such as almonds, walnuts, or pistachios, provide a satisfying crunch and healthy fats.

5. Spice it Up: Flavor Infusions

Enhance the flavor of your sugar-free desserts by incorporating aromatic spices such as cinnamon, nutmeg, or cardamom. These additions not only elevate the taste but also create a comforting and indulgent experience. Experiment with different spice combinations to find the perfect balance that suits your palate.

Baking without refined sugar is not about sacrifice; it's about reimagining the sweet experience. By embracing natural sweeteners, fruit purees, whole grain flours, dried fruits, nuts, and aromatic spices, you can create a repertoire of sweet and healthy desserts that not only satisfy your cravings but also contribute to your overall well-being. Master the art of baking without refined sugar, and enjoy the delicious journey towards a healthier and more mindful dessert experience.

Conclusion

The Pritikin Diet Cookbook stands as a testament to the harmonious fusion of health and culinary delight. By adhering to the principles of the Pritikin Diet, this cookbook has opened a door to a world of nutritious, delicious, and sustainable eating. The emphasis on whole, unprocessed foods, lean proteins, and high-fiber carbohydrates not only promotes weight management but also supports overall cardiovascular health and well-being.

Through a diverse array of recipes, the cookbook demonstrates that wholesome eating need not sacrifice flavor. From vibrant salads to hearty main courses and delectable desserts, each dish is a celebration of fresh, natural ingredients and mindful preparation.

Furthermore, the Pritikin Diet Cookbook serves as a practical guide, offering not only a collection of recipes but also insights into the science behind the diet. Readers are empowered with knowledge about the impact of food choices on their health, enabling them to make informed decisions that resonate with the Pritikin philosophy.

In an era where dietary choices play a pivotal role in our well-being, the Pritikin Diet Cookbook emerges as a valuable resource. It encourages a shift towards a lifestyle marked by balance, sustainability, and culinary pleasure without compromising on health. As individuals embark on their journey to better eating habits, this cookbook serves as a trusted companion, inviting them to savor the goodness of nutritious, delicious meals that nourish the body and delight the palate.

www.ingramcontent.com/pod-product-compliance
Lightning Source LLC
Chambersburg PA
CBHW070856260726
48661CB00004B/1433